Epsom Salt Remedies

30+ Homemade Recipes for Your Health And Body

All photos used in this book, including the cover photo were made available under a Attribution 2.0 Generic (CC BY 2.0) and sourced from Flickr

Table of Contents

Introduction 3
Chapter 1 – Significance of Epsom salt 5
   Benefits of Epsom salt 5
Chapter 2 – Epsom salt – a source of good health 8
Chapter 3 – Recipes of Epsom salt for improving health and body 11
Chapter 4 – Epsom salt for losing your weight 22
Chapter 5 – Epsom salt for enhancing your beauty 35
Conclusion 44

Introduction

Epsom salt is that mineral compound which is mostly found in the framework of gems that delicately helps in making your skin smoother if your skin has become dried. Consistently utilized by a developing number of models and performers, it's a well-known decision for having a health which has been upgraded. Blend it with your most loved conditioner which you use on daily basis to add volume to your hair or you can take it in to your shower to recharge the level of magnesium in your body. If you take Epsom salt, it will help you to have a relieved feeling in case of your health.

Studies demonstrate that magnesium and sulfur are the two normally happening minerals may assist plants to become greener with higher yields and more flowers. Magnesium makes a domain helpful for development by helping seeds to grow, expanding chlorophyll creation and enhancing the uptake of phosphorus and nitrogen.

Magnesium and sulfur are the two minerals which occur naturally and that are the essential components of Epsom salt. Magnesium is a basic mineral which helps in germinating the seeds. Plants use it to transfer the chlorophyll and it also helps in increasing the process of assimilation of phosphorus and nitrogen. Sulfur is additionally a key component in the development of plants, which ultimately help in producing vitamins as well. Tests by the National Gardening Association demonstrate that Epsom salt helps the plants in growing new flowers and help in making the other plants to become bigger in size.

Magnesium is found in vegetables and grains, and it has been an important part of all the fruits and vegetables which you take in daily routine. However numerous muds are magnesium inadequate either normally or because of over trimming. Magnesium is additionally found in ocean water. It is vital to life and you can avoid many kind of diseases if you opt for using Epsom salt in your daily routine.

Studies have demonstrated that magnesium and sulfate are both promptly absorbed with the help of skin, and this makes the Epsom salt showers a simple and perfect approach to appreciate s many medical advantages which have been associated with it.

Chapter 1 – Significance of Epsom salt

The advantages which are associated with Epsom salt are not very new to be discussed. Actually, there are so many studies that have shown the significant and wide level advantages of magnesium and sulfate, which are those minerals which are present in a large amount in the Epsom salt. So many experts, well known people, fitness instructors, and even supermodels, all have taken advantages from the use of Epsom salt.

Benefits of Epsom salt

Specialists trust that if you take shower with Epsom salt for at least three times a week then it will help you to look better, feel better and in getting high level of energy. Magnesium particles likewise unwind and make the problems lessened by bringing down the effects brought by adrenaline. They make a casual feeling and help in enhancing the rest and focus, and help your muscles and nerves to work legitimately.

An Epsom salt shower is known to be non-torment and may help in decreasing the level of irritation making it useful in the treatment of sore muscles, asthma and some kind of headaches as well. Blend a thick glue of Epsom salt with hot water and apply in order to feel high level of comfort.

If you feel tired and if your feet are having any skin problem then you are required to dip your feet in a tub of water with a large portion of some of Epsom Salt. Epsom salt helps in making your skin smoother and will even kill the smell which comes from your foot. Various studies have uncovered that Epsom salt can be utilized for an effective treatment of clogging. When it is taken inside, Epsom salt goes about as a detoxifying specialists for better purification of colon.

To get so many of the medical advantages of Epsom salt, you should take some unwinding, and anxiety elevating Epsom salt showers three times week after week by including a small amount of Epsom Salt to a hot shower and drenching for no less than 18 minutes. For the included advantage of making your skin saturated, include a container of olive oil. Try not to utilize cleanser as it will meddle with the activity of salt and attempt to rest for around two hours a short time later.

Sulfate is likewise very significant to life in a variety of ways. Sulfate is fundamental for the development of proteins in joints, additionally for digestive compounds and help in protecting the coating of gut's wall. Moreover sulfate is key to the proper alignment of cerebrum tissue and is likewise included in detoxification. Sulfate is not consumed a lot as a part of diet but it is basically used as a component of Epsom salt.

You can get the effective benefits of Epsom salt if you opt for using it on daily basis. The confirmation additionally demonstrates that the extra sulfate and magnesium are normally uprooted by the kidneys, generally as it is whether you have surplus in the eating plan or not.

It is clearly framing the examination that a percentage of the unlimited number of advantages of skimming are because of the Magnesium Sulfate itself, and these advantages can be considerable owing to the fact that they help you a lot in getting ultimate health benefits without any hurdle.

You can make effective use of Epsom salt in light of the fact that experience has demonstrated to be the best. Some Epsom salt which is present and then utilized in solid form will make your water brown in color and unusable on account of so many debasements. This is basically due to the presence of colors from metals in the water as well. This goes away following a couple of days. But sometimes the bad type of Epsom Salt is much more awful. Here is a basic test. Take an example of the proposed Epsom salt and half fill a glass tumbler. Add heated water to the top and mix until all dissolved.

Showers can be restorative and comforting if you add Epsom salt in to them. The main reason individuals take them is to wipe off the mud and stink of the whole day after getting back to home. There is nothing messy with getting a charge out of the demonstration which can be taken after having an Epsom salt shower. You can get a book, light a few candles, set out a glass of wine, and put on your most loved moderate music and can make use of Epsom salt for getting solace. You can likewise include some Epsom salt as well.

It is amazingly impossible to miss to hear that Epsom salt shower can be used to diminishing weight. As a rule, Epsom salt is used to get lightening in muscle torment. Regardless, shockingly, it is in like manner a strong answer for reducing soreness and weight. A reason for weight increment is over the top confirmation of toxins in the body. Epsom salt contains both sulfate and magnesium which to make sure clears harms and recover minor injuries.

Chapter 2 – Epsom salt – a source of good health

One of your most loved things may be to absorb an Epsom salts shower after a very hectic day of psychic or even physical work. It attempts to relieve me on all levels of body, mind and soul. Another component in decreased magnesium levels has been our accentuation on adequately getting calcium. It's a touchy move calcium debilitates magnesium yet calcium limits best when enough magnesium is accessible.

To diminish those extra creeps, include one tablespoon of Epsom salt in your washing water reliably. It is proposed that you begin with 1 tablespoon and regulated form and then add up to 1 glasses. Regardless, if you start off with some Epsom salt in the water you may experience mental scenes, crotchetiness, and hyperactivity.

To get a better smell, you can pour a few drops of any oil in it. Regardless, a couple studies suggest that extension of some distinctive fixings, for instance, oil diminishes the effect of this shower. Exactly when added to mineral water, this salt reasonably patches muscle torment. Epsom salt shower is furthermore called detox shower as it pulls out plenitude water and toxic substances from the body. People who tidy up furthermore feel uneasiness free.

Studies demonstrate that taking a calcium supplement without enough magnesium can grow the inadequacy of both supplements. Examiners have found that various Americans have five times as much calcium as magnesium in their bodies, notwithstanding the way that the most ideal extent for perfect maintenance of both minerals is two to one.

Since the magnesium from the Epsom salts is assimilated specifically in your skin, it permits even individuals who think that it is hard to take magnesium orally to have the capacity to top themselves up with this enchanted mineral.

Magnesium is an imperative component of the internal portion of our body. It is utilized by the sensory system, in addition to the utilization by our muscles. When we do psychic or some hectic physical work, we additionally consume heaps of magnesium. Magnesium is a co-variable in more than 100 catalytic activities by enzymes in the human body, for example, co-calculating with calcium to assemble and support solid bones. It gives us a high level of energy, anticipates muscle spasms and agonies, and make us to feel comfortable and solace.

Magnesium is imperative in that it keeps movement of chemicals in your body alt the way consistent, and it helps your substantial systems to run easily without having any kind of hurdle. More than half of all Americans are suffering from deficiency of magnesium, which is accepted to be an element in a wide range of issues related to health. Sulfate additionally assumes an imperative part in the path in which your body works: It has a part in the development of cerebrum tissue and joint proteins, and it can fortify the walls of directive tract.

The marvels of Epsom salt have been surely understood for a long time and not at all like different salts, has Epsom salt had valuable properties that can mitigate the body, psyche and soul. A percentage of the endless medical advantages incorporate unwinding the sensory system, curing skin issues, alleviating back agony and hurting appendages, facilitating muscle strain, recuperating cuts, treating cool and clog, and drawing poisons from the body.

If you scrub down the Epsom salt, it helps to restore magnesium and sulfate in your body on the grounds that they can be absorbed through your skin. A few specialists suggest splashing the water of Epsom salt for three times each week for around 11 to 18 minutes. In case you're pondering where to discover Epsom salt, simply look at your nearby market, or any of the drug store which is in your access easily.

Many of us consider the significance of iron and calcium for our bodies, but what do you consider magnesium? It is the second most abundant component of human cells and the fourth most basic determinedly charged molecule in the body. It helps the with body in overseeing more than 310 types and accept a basic part in masterminding various genuine limits, like muscle control, electrical inspirations, essentialness era and the transfer of damaging toxins.

Epsom salts are very much utilized by sportsmen and ladies as a cure for a lot of types of pains which they face. Notwithstanding, if you do not definitely know, Epsom salts are also very commonly used by so many celebrities as well. Gwyneth Paltrow and Victoria Beckham are known devotees of utilizing Epsom salts to get a level stomach, while so many models are said to have Epsom salt showers recently before a swimming outfit shoot to guarantee that they look and feel their best.

Many people recall Epsom Salt as an item that was in the medication bureau when they were growing up, however this item can likewise give spa-like results. A splash or shedding treatment utilizing this normally happening compound restores imperative magnesium levels in the body, decreases stretch and leaves skin brilliant and gleaming. Best of all, it costs just a couple bucks and can be found at your neighborhood drug store, market and commonly at the Dollar Store.

Epsom salt has different restorative preferences which have various fabulousness vocations. It is containing the essential compound of magnesium sulfate. Magnesium, one of the sections of human cells, is required by the body to control more than 300 mixtures and expect a crucial part in various significant limits.

Chapter 3 – Recipes of Epsom salt for improving health and body

Simply blend almost one teaspoon of Epsom salt with your most loved cleansing cream, and work the blend it into your skin, while using a round movement, to uproot dead skin cells, then wash. You'll get awesome skin with high level of smoothness.

Recipe 1

Ingredients:

- Jojoba oil six drops
- Peppermint oil 10 drops
- Ginger oil 1 drops
- Epsom salt 1 teaspoon
- Water as required

Method:

- Make a combination of all of the above mentioned ingredients.
- Avoid to contaminate it with extra drops of what has been included.
- Apply it to your skin by not adding the water or add it into the bath tub for taking bath.
- This will make your skin smoother and free of dryness.

Recipe 2

Ingredients:

- Jojoba oil six drops
- Olive oil six drops
- Lemon oil four drops
- Epsom salt 1 tablespoon
- Peppermint oil 1 drop

Method:

- Make a combination of all of the above mentioned ingredients.
- Avoid to contaminate it with extra drops of what has been included.
- Apply it to your skin by not adding the water or add it into the bath tub for taking bath.
- This will make your skin smoother and free of dryness.

Recipe 3

Ingredients:

- Rosemary oil 1 drop
- Ginger oil 1 drops
- Epsom salt 1 tablespoon
- Almond oil six drops
- Black cumin oil 3 drops

Method:

- Make a combination of all of the above mentioned ingredients.
- Avoid to contaminate it with extra drops of what has been included.
- Apply it to your skin by not adding the water or add it into the bath tub for taking bath.
- This will make your skin smoother and free of dryness.

Recipe 4

Ingredients:

- Vitamin e oil 7 drops
- Cumin oil 1 drops
- Olive oil 3 drops
- Epsom salt 1 tablespoon
- Spearmint oil six drops

Method:

- Make a combination of all of the above mentioned ingredients.
- Avoid to contaminate it with extra drops of what has been included.
- Apply it to your skin by not adding the water or add it into the bath tub for taking bath.
- This will make your skin smoother and free of dryness.

Recipe 5

Ingredients:

- Marjoram oil six drops
- Lemon oil 2 drops
- Epsom salt 1 tablespoon
- Ginger oil four drops

Method:

- Make a combination of all of the above mentioned ingredients.
- Avoid to contaminate it with extra drops of what has been included.
- Apply it to your skin by not adding the water or add it into the bath tub for taking bath.
- This will make your skin smoother and free of dryness.

Recipe 6

Ingredients:

- Coconut oil 1 drops
- Lavender oil six drops
- Epsom salt 1 tablespoon
- Peppermint oil seven drops
- Almond oil 1 drops

Method:

- Make a combination of all of the above mentioned ingredients.
- Avoid to contaminate it with extra drops of what has been included.
- Apply it to your skin by not adding the water or add it into the bath tub for taking bath.
- This will make your skin smoother and free of dryness.

Recipe 7

Ingredients:

- Fennel seeds oil six drops
- Laurel leaf oil 1 teaspoon
- Epsom salt 1 tablespoon
- Olive oil four teaspoon

Method:

- Make a combination of all of the above mentioned ingredients.
- Avoid to contaminate it with extra drops of what has been included.
- Apply it to your skin by not adding the water or add it into the bath tub for taking bath.
- This will make your skin smoother and free of dryness.

Recipe 8

Ingredients:

- Cinnamon oil four drops
- Rosemary essential oil 2 teaspoon
- Olive oil 1 teaspoon
- Epsom salt 1 tablespoon
- Apple cider vinegar half cup

Method:

- Make a combination of all of the above mentioned ingredients.
- Add it to your bath tub and take bath.
- This will make your skin smoother and oil will eventually disappear.

Recipe 9

Ingredients:

- Eucalyptus oil 1 teaspoon
- Peppermint oil 8 teaspoon
- Ginger oil 7 drops
- Frankincense essential oil four drops
- Lemon oil 1 teaspoon
- Fennel seeds oil four teaspoon

Method:

- Make a combination of all of the above mentioned ingredients.
- Avoid to contaminate it with extra drops of what has been included.
- Apply it to your skin by not adding the water or add it into the bath tub for taking bath.
- This will make your skin smoother and free of dryness.

Recipe 10

Ingredients:

- Olive oil 1 teaspoon
- Sage oil four drops
- Epsom salt 1 tablespoon
- Ginger oil 8 drops
- Orange peel oil 8 drops

Method:

- Make a combination of all of the above mentioned ingredients.
- Avoid to contaminate it with extra drops of what has been included.
- Apply it to your skin by not adding the water or add it into the bath tub for taking bath.
- This will make your skin smoother and free of dryness.

Recipe 11

Ingredients:

- Peppermint oil 1 teaspoon
- Lemon juice 1 drops
- Ginger oil 7 drops
- Lemon oil six drops
- Frankincense essential oil 1 drops
- Cumin oil six drops

Method:

- Make a combination of all of the above mentioned ingredients.
- Avoid to contaminate it with extra drops of what has been included.
- Apply it to your skin by not adding the water or add it into the bath tub for taking bath.
- This will make your skin smoother and free of dryness.

Chapter 4 – Epsom salt for losing your weight

Recipe 1

Ingredients:

- Jojoba oil six drops
- Olive oil 8 drops
- Epsom salt 2 tablespoon
- Lemon oil four drops
- Peppermint oil four drops

Method:

- Make a mixture of all the above mentioned ingredients.
- Apply it to your body from where you want to shed the extra fats.
- Massage gently twice or thrice a week for getting highly effective results.

Recipe 2

Ingredients:

- Grapefruit oil six drops
- Olive oil four drops
- Sweet almond oil 7 drops
- Epsom salt 2 tablespoon
- Cinnamon oil four drops

Method:

- Make a mixture of all the above mentioned ingredients.
- Apply it to your body from where you want to shed the extra fats.
- Massage gently twice or thrice a week for getting highly effective results.

Recipe 3

Ingredients:

- Epsom salt 2 tablespoon
- Peppermint oil six drops
- Almond oil 8 drops
- Ginger oil 1 drops
- Olive oil 3 drops

Method:

- Make a mixture of all the above mentioned ingredients.
- Apply it to your body from where you want to shed the extra fats.
- Massage gently twice or thrice a week for getting highly effective results.

Recipe 4

Ingredients:

- Nutmeg oil six drops
- Rosemary oil four drops
- Epsom salt 2 tablespoon
- Ginger oil 1 drops
- Almond oil four drops
- Black cumin oil four drops

Method:

- Make a mixture of all the above mentioned ingredients.
- Apply it to your body from where you want to shed the extra fats.
- Massage gently twice or thrice a week for getting highly effective results.

Recipe 5

Ingredients:

- Basil oil four drops
- Almond oil six drops
- Epsom salt 2 tablespoon
- Jojoba oil 1 drops
- Lemon oil six drops

Method:

- Make a mixture of all the above mentioned ingredients.
- Apply it to your body from where you want to shed the extra fats.
- Massage gently twice or thrice a week for getting highly effective results.

Recipe 6

Ingredients:

- Peppermint oil 8 drops
- Epsom salt 2 tablespoon
- Cilantro oil 3 drops

Method:

- Make a mixture of all the above mentioned ingredients.
- Apply it to your body from where you want to shed the extra fats.
- Massage gently twice or thrice a week for getting highly effective results.

Recipe 7

Ingredients:

- Cinnamon oil 7 drops
- Anise oil four drops
- Epsom salt 2 tablespoon
- Olive oil four drops
- Corn mint oil 8 drops

Method:

- Make a mixture of all the above mentioned ingredients.
- Apply it to your body from where you want to shed the extra fats.
- Massage gently twice or thrice a week for getting highly effective results.

Recipe 8

Ingredients:

- Vitamin e oil six drops
- Epsom salt 2 tablespoon
- Cumin oil 7 drops
- Olive oil 8 drops
- Spearmint oil six drops

Method:

- Make a mixture of all the above mentioned ingredients.
- Apply it to your body from where you want to shed the extra fats.
- Massage gently twice or thrice a week for getting highly effective results.

Recipe 9

Ingredients:

- Peppermint oil four drops
- Olive oil four drops
- Epsom salt 2 tablespoon
- Cumin oil 7 drops
- Almond oil 4 drops

Method:

- Make a mixture of all the above mentioned ingredients.
- Apply it to your body from where you want to shed the extra fats.
- Massage gently twice or thrice a week for getting highly effective results.

Recipe 10

Ingredients:

- Lavender oil 7 drops
- Peppermint oil 3 drops
- Epsom salt 2 tablespoon
- Frankincense essential oil 1 drops
- Ginger oil 4 drops
- Olive oil 6 drops

Method:

- Make a mixture of all the above mentioned ingredients.
- Apply it to your body from where you want to shed the extra fats.
- Massage gently twice or thrice a week for getting highly effective results.

Recipe 11

Ingredients:

- Olive oil 3 drops
- Cumin oil 8 drops
- Epsom salt 2 tablespoon
- Grapefruit oil 1 drops

Method:

- Make a mixture of all the above mentioned ingredients.
- Apply it to your body from where you want to shed the extra fats.
- Massage gently twice or thrice a week for getting highly effective results.

Recipe 12

Ingredients:

- Basil oil 7 drops
- Almond oil 1 drops
- Epsom salt 1 tablespoon
- Nutmeg oil 1 drops
- Rosemary oil six drops
- Ginger oil 8 drops

Method:

- Make a mixture of all the above mentioned ingredients.
- Apply it to your body from where you want to shed the extra fats.
- Massage gently twice or thrice a week for getting highly effective results.

Recipe 13

Ingredients:

- Peppermint oil 8 drops
- Cilantro oil 3 drops
- Olive oil four drops
- Epsom salt 1 tablespoon
- Cumin oil 8 drops
- Almond oil 1 drops

Method:

- Make a mixture of all the above mentioned ingredients.
- Apply it to your body from where you want to shed the extra fats.
- Massage gently twice or thrice a week for getting highly effective results.

Chapter 5 – Epsom salt for enhancing your beauty

Recipe 1

Ingredients:

- Jojoba oil six drops
- Almond oil four drops
- Cinnamon oil four drops
- Lemon oil 3 drops
- Epsom salt 2 tablespoon

Method:

- Make a mixture of all the ingredients which have been mentioned above.
- Allow it to rest for some time.
- Then add it to the bottle of glass or plastic as per your convenience.
- Apply it to your skin by adding it to any of the skin care cream or you can also apply it to your skin directly.
- This will help you in enhancing your beauty by bringing back the softness of your skin.

Recipe 2

Ingredients:

- Marjoram oil 8 drops
- Lemon oil 8 drops
- Ginger oil 3 drops
- Epsom salt 2 tablespoon

Method:

- Make a mixture of all the ingredients which have been mentioned above.
- Allow it to rest for some time.
- Then add it to the bottle of glass or plastic as per your convenience.
- Apply it to your skin by adding it to any of the skin care cream or you can also apply it to your skin directly.
- This will help you in enhancing your beauty by bringing back the softness of your skin.

Recipe 3

Ingredients:

- Coconut oil four teaspoon
- Epsom salt 2 tablespoon
- Avocado oil 1 teaspoon
- Lavender essential oil four teaspoon
- Dill seed oil four drops

Method:

- Make a mixture of all the ingredients which have been mentioned above.
- Allow it to rest for some time.
- Then add it to the bottle of glass or plastic as per your convenience.
- Apply it to your skin by adding it to any of the skin care cream or you can also apply it to your skin directly.
- This will help you in enhancing your beauty by bringing back the softness of your skin.

Recipe 4

Ingredients:

- Black pepper oil four drops
- Epsom salt 2 tablespoon
- Rosemary essential oil six drops
- Peppermint oil 8 drops
- Olive oil four drops

Method:

- Make a mixture of all the ingredients which have been mentioned above.
- Allow it to rest for some time.
- Then add it to the bottle of glass or plastic as per your convenience.
- Apply it to your skin by adding it to any of the skin care cream or you can also apply it to your skin directly.
- This will help you in enhancing your beauty by bringing back the softness of your skin.

Recipe 5

Ingredients:

- Coconut oil six drops
- Lavender oil four drops
- Peppermint oil four drops
- Epsom salt 2 tablespoon
- Almond oil 7 drops

Method:

- Make a mixture of all the ingredients which have been mentioned above.
- Allow it to rest for some time.
- Then add it to the bottle of glass or plastic as per your convenience.
- Apply it to your skin by adding it to any of the skin care cream or you can also apply it to your skin directly.
- This will help you in enhancing your beauty by bringing back the softness of your skin.

Recipe 6

Ingredients:

- Cumin seed oil six drops
- Dill weed oil four drops
- Olive oil 8 drops
- Epsom salt 2 tablespoon
- Lemon oil 8 drops
- Ginger oil four drops

Method:

- Make a mixture of all the ingredients which have been mentioned above.
- Allow it to rest for some time.
- Then add it to the bottle of glass or plastic as per your convenience.
- Apply it to your skin by adding it to any of the skin care cream or you can also apply it to your skin directly.
- This will help you in enhancing your beauty by bringing back the softness of your skin.

Recipe 7

Ingredients:

- Olive oil 8 drops
- Cumin oil 3 drops
- Basil oil four drops
- Bitter almond oil 8 drops
- Epsom salt 2 tablespoon
- Rosemary essential oil six drops

Method:

- Make a mixture of all the ingredients which have been mentioned above.
- Allow it to rest for some time.
- Then add it to the bottle of glass or plastic as per your convenience.
- Apply it to your skin by adding it to any of the skin care cream or you can also apply it to your skin directly.
- This will help you in enhancing your beauty by bringing back the softness of your skin.

Recipe 8

Ingredients:

- Fennel seeds oil six drops
- Laurel leaf oil 1 teaspoon
- Epsom salt 2 tablespoon
- Olive oil 1 teaspoon
- Coconut essential oil 8 teaspoon
- Ginger essential oil 8 drops

Method:

- Make a mixture of all the ingredients which have been mentioned above.
- Allow it to rest for some time.
- Then add it to the bottle of glass or plastic as per your convenience.
- Apply it to your skin by adding it to any of the skin care cream or you can also apply it to your skin directly.
- This will help you in enhancing your beauty by bringing back the softness of your skin.

Recipe 9

Ingredients:

- Rose essential oil four drops
- Olive oil 1 drop
- Ginger essential oil 3 drops
- Epsom salt 2 tablespoon
- Cumin oil 8 drops
- Savory oil 8 drops

Method:

- Make a mixture of all the ingredients which have been mentioned above.
- Allow it to rest for some time.
- Then add it to the bottle of glass or plastic as per your convenience.
- Apply it to your skin by adding it to any of the skin care cream or you can also apply it to your skin directly.
- This will help you in enhancing your beauty by bringing back the softness of your skin.

Conclusion

Epsom Salt is magnesium sulfate. It offers a standout among the best methods for making your body needs of magnesium accessible in an effective way. Abundance of adrenaline and anxiety are known to deplete the level of magnesium, an item which can relieve some sort of characteristic anxiety from the body. Magnesium is fundamental for the body to tie sufficient measures of serotonin, a state of mind hoisting concoction inside of the cerebrum that makes a sentiment prosperity and brings you comfort.

Scientists and doctors report that raising your magnesium levels may help in enhancing the health of heart and circulatory system, decrease sporadic heartbeats, avoid blockage of the veins, decrease the clusters of blood and lower pulse followed by enhancing the capacity of body to utilize insulin, decreasing the occurrence or seriousness of diabetes. Epsom salt additionally conveys sulfates, which are to a great degree hard to overcome nourishment yet which promptly assimilate through the skin.

Medicinal examination demonstrates sulfates are required for the development of mind tissue, joint proteins and the mucin proteins that line the digestive's dividers tract. Sulfates additionally fortify the pancreas to produce digestive chemicals and detoxify the body's deposit of solutions and ecological contaminants.

FREE Bonus Reminder

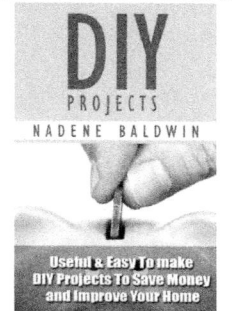

If you have not grabbed it yet, please go ahead and download your special bonus report *"DIY Projects. 13 Useful & Easy To Make DIY Projects To Save Money & Improve Your Home!"*
Simply Click the Button Below

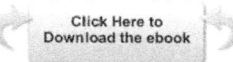

OR **Go to This Page**
http://diyhomecraft.com/free

BONUS #2: More Free Books
Do you want to receive more Free Books?
We have a mailing list where we send out our new Books when they go free on Kindle. Click on the link below to sign up for Free Book Promotions.
=> Sign Up for Free Book Promotions <=

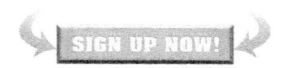

OR Go to this URL
http://zbit.ly/1WBb1Ek

Printed in Great Britain
by Amazon